Dementia Activities

Keeping Occupied and Stimulated
Can Improve Their Quality of Life

By

Natalie Johnson

Table of Contents

Introduction

Thank you for purchasing this eBook. You are now on a path towards learning about how to improve the quality of life for people suffering from dementia. There are over 5 million people in the United States and 1 million people in the United Kingdom that suffer from dementia.

It is a condition that affects both the rich and the poor, but mostly older people over 65 years of age. There is no cure for dementia and those who suffer from it simply have to cope with the symptoms the best way they can.

The quick and easy treatment is to take anti-dementia prescription medications because they have been known to increase people's behaviors and psychology for the better. However, they only provide temporary relief from the symptoms of dementia. There are still other emotional symptoms that develop because of dementia, which are depression, anxiety and stress. These are symptoms that any normal person would feel after their ability to live their daily life has been limited.

The only difference is that the symptoms of depression are much more severe with dementia sufferers suffering from these limitations.

This book emphasizes the importance of implementing activities into the daily lives of dementia patients. This is a natural treatment that actually works more effectively than any medications or surgeries ever could. Even though it won't make a person totally regain their brain function, it will still give them more positive feedings of independence and self worth.

These are things that go away with dementia patients because they are so used to having everyone else do things for them. While you read this book, you will learn the importance of giving patients their independence and the type of activities that they should do to achieve it. There are different levels of severity with dementia and you need to know which activities are suitable with each level. All of this will be discussed and more. But first, you must understand and learn more about dementia.

Chapter 1 - What is Dementia?

The first thing you have to understand is what dementia actually is. Some people think of it as a disease that hits older people. The truth is that dementia is not a disease, but rather a group of symptoms that make up a health condition. So when we say somebody has dementia, we are describing a condition that is negatively affecting their health. The symptoms of dementia are ones that affect the function and thinking ability of the brain. These include memory lapses, poor judgment, difficulty speaking, and constant disorientation. People like this often have trouble taking care of themselves or performing everyday routines like eating, dressing or showering.

People who suffer from dementia often get it from an actual disease, like Alzheimer's disease. There is no scientific reason why certain people get this disease and the cause of it is unknown. The only thing we know is that it usually develops in older people more than anyone else. Alzheimer's destroys their brain cells and increases their risks of getting brain damage or other negative health affects in the brain. However, dementia doesn't just automatically develop in people who get Alzheimer's disease. The dementia condition forms after the other symptoms of Alzheimer's disease take affect, which include lack of oxygen to the brain, stroke and brain trauma. If the brain endures these kinds of hardships, dementia is likely going to follow.

There are different kinds of dementia as well as diseases that cause it. These include vascular dementia, lewy body dementia, alcohol dementia and Pick's disease. All of these conditions kill brain cells. The level of severity of the damage depends on which areas of the brain are actually being attacked. Chances are you won't know you have dementia until the signs kick in. The early stages of dementia will cause you to have light memory loss, such as forgetting what time of day it is or not remembering how to find places you are familiar with. When it gets to the point where you can't remember how to get back home, then you are definitely suffering from dementia. If you experience these symptoms or know somebody who does, help must be sought after right away before the condition gets worse.

People often get confused about the symptoms of dementia. They see them as some kind of personality disorder or mental illness because the symptoms are very much alike. People with dementia or mental illness will both experience anxiety, social inappropriateness, compulsive behavior, depression and more. However, mental illness and personality disorders are caused by traumatic experiences in the past, which make someone act and behave in a way that is uncontrollable. There is nothing necessary wrong with their brain cells, but there is just deep rooted problems with their personality and behavior patterns. There is no underlying disease that is causing it, like with dementia. So be on the lookout for those differences when self diagnosing yourself or a loved one with dementia.

Chapter 2 – Three Stages of Severity

It would be wrong to treat everybody with dementia the same way because there are three different stages of severity for the condition. That is why when you try to get patients to perform certain activities, you have to make sure you know which stage of dementia they are faced with before giving them an activity to do. If you give them an activity they are unable to do, then it will make them feel worse. This is what you don't want to happen because the whole point of making them perform activities is to enhance their self confidence and make them happier. So you need to understand what these three stages of dementia are, and the specific symptoms that occur with each one. Then you can feel confident in giving them an activity that you know they can handle based on their condition.

The Mild Stage
The mild stage of dementia is the very first stage in the condition. This should be the stage when family and friends start noticing that their loved one is suffering from this condition. It will begin when a person can't find the right words to complete their sentences or the thoughts they are trying to convey onto others. The story they try to tell will sound scrambled and their recollection of the events they experienced will be a blur to them. Now you might think these are symptoms that anyone might have. After all, how many times have you tried remembering an event and you

forget some of the details you experienced? It happens all the time and it doesn't mean people are suffering from dementia. That is why it can be hard to identify the condition during the mild stage. However, there are other symptoms to lookout for in this stage. One might be the repetitiveness of them asking questions over and over again to family members who have already answered their questions. The person could also suffer from paranoia and start accusing people of doing horrible things they didn't really do.

The Moderate Stage

At this point, the symptoms of dementia should have already been identified in the person who showed the signs described in the first stage. However, it is possible they could have gotten overlooked if the person in question has a history for being forgetful or stuttering with their words. Some people just have bad short term memory, so it is easy to confuse the two conditions. But in the moderate stage, the signs of dementia will start to become much more noticeable and there will be no confusing the situation at this point. For example, the person won't be able to understand you when you talk fast or tell a long story. They will likely take a long time to respond to simple questions or to participate in conversations. Then when they do talk, they will not be as polite as they used to be. Dementia sort of erases people's ability to stay civil and polite during social situations. This means you can expect to hear random swearing, obscenities and just impolite comments to people who did nothing to provoke them.

The Severe Stage
The severe stage is when a person cannot function properly or take care of themselves because their dementia symptoms won't allow them to. Hopefully, the person already has a professional caregiver watching over them and monitoring their activities. Those in the severe stage will be people who hardly speak at all. In fact, you will be lucky to get five words out of them throughout the entire day. When they do talk they will start saying things that make no sense. Their main form of communication will be through nonverbal behaviors such as sounds or facial expressions. Unfortunately, it will be hard for a caregiver to understand the message that the patient is trying to convey with these nonverbal communication attempts. But once the caregiver gets used to their patient then they will start to understand their own unique way of communicating and what their nonverbal actions are all about. In return, some patients may even be quicker to respond to nonverbal communication that comes from something or someone else. Such examples include sound, music or touch.

There is one form of nonverbal communication that should be avoided, and that is the television. If you look at modern television shows, there is so much visual variety and stimulation coming from it that it can be unhealthy for a dementia patient. All it takes is for them to see one disturbing image and it could throw them off into a physical or emotional outburst. Instead, provide more books for the patient to read or let them listen to their favorite music. The point is to make the patient as comfortable as possible without any negative triggers around that could set them off in a rage. Since television is so unpredictable with the content that is being shown on it, you don't want to take a chance of a severely disturbed dementia patient being exposed to these random images.

Activity Integration

If you are a family member of a patient or even their caregiver, you will need a doctor to truly classify what stage of severity their dementia is at. It can be hard for a layman person to figure this out because the symptoms look similar throughout all the stages of dementia. The first thing you have to remember is to try and let the patient decide on the activity first. You can politely show them a list of activities or make suggestions as to what they can do. But let them make the choice on their own, or else they will feel pushed. If they are unable to communicate their choice, then you will have to take it slow. Try implementing some of the easier activities, like watching game shows or listening to music. Then as they begin to adapt to those activities, you can try to integrate more intense activities into their lives. You'll want to get to a point where they get to doing physical activity or at least as much as they are able to do.

Caregivers will have a tougher time than family members to get a patient to participate in activities. After all, the caregiver is a stranger to them. Dementia patients are not very adaptive to anything or anyone that is new to them. That is why there is so much emphasis on getting patients to think about the past or get distracted from the present. If they have to face new things in the present then it will cause them to outburst with emotion. Therefore, if you are a caregiver then you may have to become friends with the patient before they actually trust you enough to coordinate their activities. It may be hard at first to become their friends, but after weeks and months go by they won't consider you a stranger anymore. They will consider you a friend and will listen to what you have to say. Then you can start integrating activities into their lives.

Chapter 3 - Importance of Activities

All people need activities in their lives in order to relieve their boredom and overcome their frustrations. Healthy people are able to coordinate their own activities to help do this, but dementia patients are not able to. They need help from caregivers to give them activities that they are able to do in order to make them feel self sufficient again. This is really the only treatment available for dementia patients because there are no cures or surgeries that will take the condition away. As for the main cause of the condition, Alzheimer's disease also has no cure. Therefore, the only treatments available are coping mechanisms like hobbies, activities and communication.

When providing care for dementia patients it can be very challenging because of their poor state of mind. That is why it is important that you develop daily routines and activities for them to participate in because it will distract them from the negative conditions they are living with. More importantly, it will make their lives interesting again and that will make them happy. The activities you develop for a dementia patient should fulfill all of their spiritual, physical, social and mental needs. These are the needs of all people, so by fulfilling these needs for dementia patients then they will start feeling happy again. A person's social needs are simple enough. Get them into activities where they spend time around people, like family and friends. Physical needs come along the lines of exercise activities and manual labor they do by themselves. Spiritual activities come along the lines of creativity and religion. Perhaps, the patient could go to church or create a new piece of artwork from an image in their heads. All of these together will fulfill their final need, which is mental.

The activities you develop for these needs can be quite complex because the symptoms of each dementia patient have different stages of severity. Some patients may only have minor memory issues while others could be totally out of touch with reality. So, it is crucial that you develop activities specifically catered to each individual's needs. Then as their condition gets worse, which it most often does, you will have to change their activities again to accommodate their new condition and state of mind. But in order for this to actually happen, caregivers and families both need to work together to make it happen. As you read on in this book, you will learn about a variety of different activities that work well with dementia patients. However, read the description of the activities carefully, so you can determine if they are suitable for your particular patient's condition. And always, seek the advice of a medical professional before the patient actually performs the activity. If they already have a caregiver who is a registered nurse or other health professional, then their advice will be fine.

The real importance of activities comes from the distraction they provide. If you leave a dementia patient alone in a room all day then they will look at themselves in the mirror and not like what they see. Activities are a distraction from the pain and suffering they are going through in the present. Now contrary to popular belief, it is not always a good thing to focus on the present when it comes to a person's mental state. This is especially true if the person has an incurable condition like dementia and has no hope of ever getting their old life back again. For someone like this, they either have two choices. They can die or they can live. If they choose to live then there are plenty of ways for them to find happiness, like by participating in activities. As a caregiver or loved one, you need to constantly remind the patient they have reasons to live. It is those that have nobody who choose to give up on life all together and just die. Don't let this happen to your loved one. Make sure they know you are there for them and will do whatever it takes to give them a happy life. This is the best thing we can do for anyone really.

Chapter 4 – Activities

There are four categories of activities that can fulfill a dementia patient's needs, which are self-care, work, rest and leisure activities. If you maintain a balance amongst these four areas then it will reduce their stress levels and give them more self confidence. However, the activity that is most important is work. If you look at the lifestyle of a retiree, they are often looking for something to do to fill that gap of not working. Sometimes it can even depress them by not having anything to do, whether they suffer from dementia or not. But for those who do suffer, their depression is even worse because they feel like they don't have a choice anymore. So you need to give patients chores or duties in order to fulfill their work needs. These could be simple things like paying the bills, making phone calls, dusting the furniture or doing the laundry. These all represent activities they used to do, but can still do again with a little help. If a family member or caregiver is there, they can always supervise the patient to make sure they are doing the activities correctly.

Self-care is a need that should not be neglected by anyone. The activities that make up self-care are ones that allow the patient to take care of themselves, their bodies and their home environment. This includes activities like going to the bathroom, dressing, grooming, feeding, and bathing. Since dementia patients often suffer from short term memory loss, they don't remember if they did things like brushing their teeth or taking their medication. A caregiver should leave written reminders around the home for the patient, which tells them they either accomplished these things or did not accomplish them. In a way, the caregiver will be acting as the patient's short term memory by reassuring them they did these self-care activities. The caregiver cannot push too hard on these issues though. Patients often have physical and emotional outbursts towards their caregivers who try to perform these activities for them. Caregivers are only trying to help, but over helping can lead to injuries or a refusal by the patient to do any activities. This is something that could have a profoundly negative effect on their already diminishing emotional state. That is why self-care activities need to be solely done by the patient. The caregiver is only there to encourage the patient to take care of themselves or remind them that they didn't do a certain activity, like eating or grooming.

Leisure activities are very important on so many levels. For one thing, they are one of the few times that patients actually get to have fun and enjoy themselves. They are also the one type of activity that patients want to do, instead of feeling like they have to do it. Not only that, but they help distract patients from their condition and let them focus on the creative side of their brains as well. Leisure activities could be a variety of things. The most popular one is jigsaw puzzles, board games and card games. For those patients who have an artistic side to them, they could paint pictures, write stories, play instruments or any other artistic quality they possess.

Dementia Activities

Dementia doesn't necessarily erase the skills and talents that patients have adapted throughout their lives. If you give them a chance to perform these activities then it will allow them to feel complete again by doing the one thing they love. In fact, artistic works have always been classified as ways of communication and expressionism.

However, you may come across a few patients that are a little more stubborn about leisurely activities. You have to understand that a lot of people from older generations were taught that leisure time was just a time to be lazy or unproductive. The only type of leisurely activity these people know is socializing, like at a lunch or friendly meeting. So for these kinds of people, try to get their family and friends to visit them as often as possible. Everybody has some activity that brings them joy and distracts them from their own lives. Socializing is the one activity that every generation has adapted, so it should almost always work for your dementia patient.

Depending on the level of dementia, caregivers should try to refrain from actually doing the work for them. Instead, they should only coordinate the chores and try to make the patient feel like they are really necessary, instead of just something that is meant to help their condition. Dementia patients may be slow mentally, but they have not lost all of their intelligence. If you start treating them like a mental patient who can't do anything for themselves, then they will pick up on that fast and get depressed. You have to remember that just because they suffer from dementia doesn't mean they are totally ignorant and stupid. Dementia patients still have lots of memories and recollections still left in their brains. As a caregiver, you are just there to help them fill the gaps that are stopping them from being whole again.

List of Activities

Exercise – No matter what state of mind a person is in, it is always crucial that they get their exercise in order to maintain their physical health. After all, a healthy body helps create a healthy mind and vice versa. The real trick here is to find an exercise that is suitable for each particular dementia patient, since the severity of their symptoms could be different. Now the easiest exercise for anyone to do is walking. This is a low intensity cardiovascular exercise that won't strain the body, but will get a person's heart beating and blood flowing. If long distances are a problem then they can take short walks around the block under a caregiver's supervision, of course. It is always good to make walking a daily routine that is set at a specific time every day. The consistency of the scheduled walking each day will help them to remember to do it on their own. With all the physical exertion, they will even have an easier time getting to sleep at time and their minds won't wander as much in their imagination. Please note that the caregiver should make sure the patient is dressed appropriately for the weather conditions outside because those are subject to change and the patient may not have the brain function to adapt to the changing weather conditions on their own. More specific exercises will be discussed as you move down the list of activities.

Dogs & Cats – There is a good reason why so many people are pet owners. A dog or cat can light up a person's life, especially if they have nobody else in it. In fact, do you ever notice how people who have suffered a traumatic experience get exposed to dogs as a form of therapeutic treatment? There is something about the innocence and loving nature of pets that brighten up a person's life. Dementia patients feel alone and awkward
around people because of their mental state. The great thing about pets is they don't judge or criticize anyone. So by having a dementia patient play with pets or even walk them, they will feel like they have a new friend to hang around with during their tough situation.

Community – A community full of people is a good thing for a dementia patient to take part in. If they get involved with community activities, like church or bingo, it will allow them to get out more and see friends they don't normally see. Also, if the patient is in a special community filled with other patients who have similar conditions, then they will feel more secure about going out in public and socializing with the people around them. They can share their experiences with each other and try to gain support from them. It is almost like going to an A.A. meeting where the alcoholics share their stories with each other to better cope with their own situation. Dementia patients who still have the capacity to communicate will benefit greatly from this. As for the ones who have trouble communicating, they can still benefit from listening to other dementia patients and feel comfortable being around them because of their similarities.

Music – It is pretty safe to say that music is something everyone enjoys. The only difference is that we all have our own preferences when it comes to the kind of music we like to listen to. For dementia patients, it can be greatly beneficial for them to hear music that reminds them of happier times in their lives. It can be soft music that is relaxing and helps them take their mind off their condition. The best part is that music can be played anywhere these days. You can get them a mobile device, such as a walkman, that has all their favorite songs loaded into it or on a disc. You could try getting them an iPod or even a Smartphone for the music, but older people who didn't grow up with this technology will have a tougher time getting it to work. Even people who are in their 40s and 50s have trouble working these gadgets, so anyone older who has dementia will probably have great difficulty with it. That is why getting them a walkman that holds cassettes might be the best option because it is something from their youth that they are more familiar with.

If the patient is able to sing and dance, then that would be even better because it would involve more physical activity. It is also one of the few physical activities that can be done right in the comfort of their own home. Believe it or not, many people who have moderate and severe dementia are still able to communicate through the power of singing and dancing. What's even better is if the person plays an instrument that they used to play when they were younger. Remember that skills like these stay with patients throughout their lives. Music, singing, dancing and playing instruments are all things that will help patients relive their youth and remind them of happier times. As a caregiver, your job is simply to give them the opportunity to let this happen. This means you provide the music, the walkman and the instruments they need to make it happen.

Massage – A massage is more of an activity that is being done to patients, but it is one that will give them a great sense of relaxation. It also allows the caregiver and patient to form a personal bond, which will develop a sense of trust in the patient for their caregiver. This is important for so many reasons, especially with communication. Once the severity of the patient's dementia has gotten worse, they won't be able to communicate verbally anymore. So if a caregiver has been giving their patient massages for awhile, then the patient will develop a sense of trust for the caregiver and won't give them such a hard time when the dementia gets worse.

Reading – If a dementia patient is still able to read, then this is the perfect leisurely distraction away from the condition. It is also for exercising the brain because the patient will have to use their imagination more when reading stories from a book. However, there are some dementia patients that will have trouble reading because their mental illness has limited their ability to concentrate on one thing at a time. So if they go to read a book, newspaper or magazine, they could lose interest within minutes if their lack of concentration causes their mind to wander to other places. If a caregiver comes across such a patient, they should read the material out loud for the patient because verbal speech is easier for them to focus on then written text. Then they can get caught up on world news and events. If the patient gets visits from their friends and family, then they can assist with the reading as well.

Audio books may be an alternative that a dementia patient can take advantage of if they don't have anyone to read to them. It also enhances their sense of independence because they can listen to the audio books by themselves anytime they want. In our modern technological age, there are dozens of places where audio books can be obtained. A caregiver can assist the patient in purchasing these audio books from places like libraries, bookshops, Amazon.com and so on. There are even some newspaper publications that now offer a newspaper talking service, which is basically like a radio show where someone reads the daily news.

Picture books should be kept around the patient's house for them to look at anytime they want. Since they may have trouble reading, pictures are a visual alternative that helps stimulate their brain faster and requires less concentration on their part. They can easily remember images from a picture book and still feel like they read a story. Just make sure the picture book is pleasant material that will make them feel good inside.

Some Television – As you read on in this book, you will learn that television is not recommended for dementia patients because of the random amounts of images they will encounter. More than likely, they will end up encountering an image that will disturb them and then cause an outburst. However, if you have parental controls over their television then you can set the controls to television shows that are more stimulating to their mind. These could be game shows, quiz shows, old films or documentaries. Just make sure they are programs that get the patient to think and use their brains. If you start showing them Rambo movies that has constant death and violence, then you are going to make them feel anxious and scared.

Now if you are not able to control the programs that come on the television for your patient, try playing DVDs or videos that have suitable content for them to watch. You can just completely get rid of any cable service they have, and instead buy them a DVD player with a bunch of educational DVDs. Then they can just watch those anytime they want, which will also enhance their feeling of independence.

Cooking – Patients who are in the mild to moderate stages of dementia will likely still have the mental capacity to cook their own meals. The importance of cooking is that it can help trigger old memories in the patient of a time when they used to cook meals for themselves. So if you have them cook the meals they know how to make then they will start remembering more of their past. However, if they are trying to cook meals based on new recipes they have never tried before, then they will need assistance. Depending on the severity of the patient's dementia, they may not be able to read the recipes from a cookbook. Therefore, they will need assistance in reading the recipes and gathering the ingredients.

The great thing about cooking activities is that they make the patient feel independent, but at the same time cooking can be a two person job. This gives the caregiver an excuse to be the patient's assistant in the kitchen and help them out with preparing the recipes. This is especially important if the patient has severe dementia because they will be held back a lot by their limitations. In fact, it is better that severe dementia patients cook foods that are super easy to prepare or are easily familiar. For example, let's say it is Thanksgiving and the patient wants to cook a turkey with mashed potatoes, stuffing and gravy. This is a very familiar meal that they have probably cooked every year of their lives, so they will have the recipe and knowledge in their head on how to prepare it.

Another great idea for assisting dementia patients in the kitchen is by having them give you orders. You can pretend that you don't know how to cook the meal being prepared and that you need them to tell you. This makes the patient feel important and will actually boost their ego by making them feel like they are in charge. Now if for some reason they tell you the wrong directions, don't be so quick to judge them as being wrong. Instead, have a recipe book nearby that states how to cook the meal properly. So if they end up giving the wrong directions, you can politely refer back to the cookbook and tell them that it states to do something different in there.

Dementia Activities

This should help them change their minds while still giving them a sense of superiority at the same time.

Bingo – This activity is most commonly associated with older people. If you have ever been to Bingo night at a church then you will see 90% of the people there are over the age of 60. Not only that, but many of them have brain diseases and the condition of dementia caused by them. So have you ever wondered why so many older people love to play Bingo? Could it be the thrill of trying to win a cash prize? To them it may be, but for their caregivers it is something else entirely. Bingo is a magnificent brain exercise that gets patients to constantly use their brain function to search for numbers on their bingo cards. That is why you see these older people with about 30 different bingo cards for one game. Every time a number is called, they are quickly scanning their eyes over all the boards trying to find their number. At the same time, it enhances their attention span and thinking ability. Bingo can also be a nice social environment because there are lots of older people with similar conditions of dementia, so the patient won't feel out of place there.

Games – We have already covered that Bingo is a great game, but there are a variety of smaller games that patients can play in the comfort of their own homes with friends. The important thing to remember is that games help dementia patients use their minds and enhances their problem solving skills. Such games include dominoes, card games, jigsaw puzzles and Scrabble. With jigsaw puzzles, you might want to get the kind that use bigger puzzle pieces because they are easier for patients to see. But try not to get any childish jigsaw puzzles that are made for kids because this will be insulting to the patient. They are still adults with real adult feelings and needs. So if you start buying them children's games or puzzles then they will likely have an emotional outburst, which you don't want to have happen.

Painting Pictures – Dementia patients are visual learners and communicators. If your patient has trouble speaking then it may be a good idea to give them a paint brush and palette, and have them paint a picture on a canvas attached to an easel. The patients don't necessarily have to be professional artists or have any particular skill as a painter. Just put the brush in their hand and watch them paint away. Sometimes this can be the only way for a patient to let out their true feelings and emotions. The picture they paint may not be perfect, but it will certainly give you an idea about what kind of thoughts are going on inside their head.

Writing – Here is an activity that can be enjoyed by those suffering from mild dementia. Their handwriting ability should still be intact, so you can encourage them to write letters to their family or perhaps even write a book about their life experiences. If they had an interesting life while they were younger, it will certainly interest them to relive those exciting times by writing them down in a book. Then who knows, you could try helping them publish the book and bring them in a bit of royalties on the side.

Clipping Coupons – Older people and those on a budget love to clip coupons because it helps them save money at the grocery store. For a dementia patient, it serves an extra purpose. It allows them to keep busy and become self dependent by helping themselves save money. A caregiver could ask the patient if they would do them a favor and clip these coupons. Since the patient wants to feel useful, they will likely be happy to oblige.

Restoring Old Furniture – This might sound like a bit of a stretch, but it has been known to work well with dementia patients. The caregivers need to buy old furniture pieces at thrift stores or garage sales, and then bring them back to the patient's home for them to fix up. This means allowing the patient to sand and polish the old furniture if they are handy with woodworking equipment. However, make sure you don't give the patient any equipment where they could harm themselves, like an electrical sander, or else they will more than likely burn themselves. Instead, give them a manual sander and a bottle of wood polish. This might take a longer time to finish the wood, but dementia patients have all the time in the world. This activity will keep them busy and make them feel special after they have successfully restored an old piece of wood into something useable again.

Thrift Store Shopping – People love to shop. It is a great way for them to just take their minds away from their troubles and look at a selection of products they don't see every day. For dementia patients, thrift stores are the best places to go because there is likely going to be older items that remind them of their youth. Thrift stores are so random and you never know what you are going to find in them. People that donate their old clothes, silverware, electronics and other goods, will likely trigger a memory in a patient's head when they see these items. Then if they want to buy the items, the prices are cheap enough to where they are affordable.

Knitting & Sewing – Older people have always been known to sew and knit as a hobby. This is more of a generational thing because people used to be taught sewing and knitting in schools, and even in the military. It was an important skill to learn because you could mend clothes with holes in them and save money from buying new ones. Therefore, you should give patients a sewing and knitting kit, so they can use their creative skills to make new clothing. Perhaps, they can knit a sweater for their grandchild and give it to them as a present on their birthday. This way they don't have to spend money they don't have or purchase an impersonal present. A hand knitted sweater has much more meaning and it will be cherished by the person who receives it. Best of all, it will make the dementia patient feel like they can still create something useful, which increases their self confidence.

Gardening – Here is an activity that everybody should take part in if they want to eat healthy foods and live a long happy life. Unfortunately, most people don't have time to garden because they work too much or simply don't know how to do it. However, older people and those suffering from dementia love gardening because it provides them with both fresh air and exercise. It also encourages them to eat healthier foods and saves them money from having to buy processed junk foods at the supermarket.

The caregiver will need to help the patient, especially if they have moderate to severe dementia. The first step is to find a spot of land around the home to start the garden on. Then the caregiver needs to dig into the soil and plant the seeds. Dementia patients will not be able to handle this kind of physical activity, which is why caregivers need to do this for them. What the patients will be able to do is the tending to the garden. This includes weeding, trimming and watering the plants. Just make sure you don't give the patient any electrical equipment because they can be dangerous for them to use. Give them a manual weed cutter for the weeding. The trimming can be done with scissors and the water comes from a hose, so that should be the easiest for them to manage. The important thing is for them to get outside around nature. The green color of the grass, plants and trees have a positive psychological affect on the human brain.

Beach Walks – This is a step up from the exercise activity. Here the caregiver will actually be taking their patient to the beach by the ocean. It is important that you choose an ocean because the water sends off negative ions into the air that people on the beach can breathe in. Negative ions are invisible molecules that are tasteless and odorless. They exist only in certain environments such as waterfalls, mountains and beaches. What happens is once you breathe in the negative ions and they enter your bloodstream, it creates a biochemical reaction that enhances your mood and makes you feel less depressed. Some say it even gives you a boost of energy as well. These are things that dementia patients so desperately need. Walking on the beach is the best way for them to get these negative ions because they have a great view, fresh air, and plenty of Vitamin D from the UV rays of the sun. The UV rays are also known to boost a person's mood.

A caregiver needs to be careful with their patient on the beach. The sand is almost always going to be uneven when you walk on it, unless you walk closer to the water where the sand is hard from the tide. Either way, the dementia patient might have trouble balancing while they walk on the sandy beach. So let them hold onto your arm while you two walk together down the beach. That way they can keep balance and inhale the negative ions at the same time.

Swimming – Lots of people with illnesses and obesity issues still enjoy swimming. It is one of the most popular exercises amongst people who are both in shape and out of shape. Dementia patients love to swim with few people in the water because they find it relaxing to swim with less distraction. Plus, this gives the caregiver a chance to monitor their patient more closely. Swimming is an exercise that only people with mild dementia should undertake. That way they will still have the mindset to stay afloat and not drown themselves.

Take a Drive – Caregivers should frequently take their patients out for a drive around town. Do not let the patient drive under any circumstances and regardless of the severity of their condition. The last thing you want to do is risk an accident that will put multiple people's lives in danger besides your patient's life. So drive them wherever they want to go. This won't necessary enhance their feeling of independence, but it will at least get them out of the house and around town.

Now you may be wondering about dementia patients that don't have caregivers, like mild stage dementia patients. If they are senior citizens then they might be entitled to free local public transportation in their town or city. Just go to city hall or the local council and ask about bus passes for older disabled individuals.

Conclusion to Activities

If have been given a lot of activities to think about here. What you need to do is write them all down on a piece of paper and then show them to the dementia patient. Have them choose a few activities that sound interesting to them. Then ask their doctor or healthcare professional if those activities are safe for them to undertake. If you have their approval then you can let the patient perform those activities.

Chapter 5 - Physical Activity

In the previous chapter, you have learned all about the various activities that a dementia patient can perform in order to enhance their quality of life. Exercises were mentioned, but it is important that you truly understand why physical activity like this is essential for their treatment. It all has to do with enhance cognitive function in the brain. There have been numerous scientific studies which have found that physical activity to be the number one treatment for those suffering from dementia or other forms of cognitive decline. This does not apply to just older people or those with dementia. This applies to the entire human race, whether you are young, middle aged or old. In fact, studies have shown people without dementia who exercise when their younger are less likely to get dementia when they are older.

Now there is no hard scientific evidence to prove why this is the case, since Alzheimer's disease and other causes of dementia are not 100% preventable. But with many of those who have gotten dementia, they were not leading physically active lives beforehand. The point is that physical activity is a natural biological need for our bodies and minds to function better as a whole. For dementia patients, they need physical activity because their brain function is continuously declining and the activity helps counterbalance it. Physical activity won't cure them, but it will slow down the decline of their brain functionality and give it more time to function properly.

Dementia patients do not have to do hours of physical exercise each day, but they should still do some form of exercise each day. The problem with many patients is they sit down for too long while lost in their thoughts. Either that or they have a disability that limits their physical activity. Well if you remember in the previous chapter, we talked about how swimming was a great exercise for those who were overweight or disabled. It allows a person to float by themselves in the water without having to use their legs. Then they can swim or even doggy paddle around the pool to get their physical exertion. The point is to get the patient out of their chair and moving around for 30 minutes per day.

Physical Activity Types
The best physical activities for dementia patients will be laid out here. Always remember to use caution when having a patient perform any of these activities because some of them require more balance and coordination than others.

Aerobics – Dementia patients need to make sure their body is taken care of as well as their mind. Aerobics, like walking and swimming, will give patients a healthy mind and a healthy body. They improve your breathing and heart rates, which keeps your lungs, blood vessels and heart at healthy conditions. Patients don't have to run marathons to get this to happen. They can take a moderate walk outside with their caregiver to as far as they want to go.

Weight Lifting – Nobody should expect a dementia patient to become Mr. Universe, but a light to moderate amount of weight lifting will do wonders for their body. But more importantly, their self esteem will fly through the roof. The main reason people get into bodybuilding in the first place has to do with self confidence and self esteem. The muscular body is just an added bonus. Since dementia patients are trying to find this confidence, weightlifting will definitely help. It will also help their bones and joints as well. Of course, they should always have a workout partner to watch them lift the weights and make sure they don't hurt themselves. This can be the caregiver if they have one.

Flexibility – These are exercises that stretch your muscles. This is very important for anyone lifting weights to do because it keeps your muscles flexible and helps prevent you from pulling muscles during a weight workout. The last thing you would want is for a dementia patient to pull their muscle because then they would have to endure that pain on top of the psychological pain they feel every day. So always do stretches before a weight or aerobic workout.

Balance Exercises – You never hear a lot of people talk about balance exercises. A lot of younger people who go to gyms never do them. For older people with dementia, they can help them stay walking and moving around by enhancing their coordination. The exercises that help with balance are yoga, tai chi, and Pilates. These exercises are recommended three times per week for older people with dementia.

Conclusion for Physical Activity

By now, you know the importance of physical activity. Just because someone has dementia doesn't mean they shouldn't perform any physical exercise. By keeping them in a confined area with no chance to move around, you are hurting them even more. Plus, the human brain has chemicals called endorphins that get released into the body during physical activity. These endorphins are meant to relax the body when it is under extreme stress or anxiety, like during a physical workout. That is why people always feel better after they go to the gym or walk around the block. The endorphins in their brain are helping them relax. Dementia patients are always under extreme stress and anxiety, so an endorphin release in their brains will help them feel better as well. So find an activity they can perform and watch how much happier they become.

Chapter 6 – Communication & Independence

Communication

People suffering from moderate or severe dementia will not be able to communicate with you verbally. Instead, behavior becomes the main source of communication for both the patient and the caregiver. The caregiver has to also use behavior as a way to communicate because the patient responds more to visual signals than verbal ones. However, this doesn't mean all patients won't understand what you say to them. The only thing is you have to keep eye contact with the patient every time you say something to them. If you talk and look away then the patient isn't going to pay attention. The caregiver must always look the patient directly in the eyes because it will help the patient focus and concentrate better. This all has to do with visual behavior. They see eyes looking at them as a signal for communication.

Dementia patients do have a few moments where they start talking, but it is usually about some experience that happened to them in the past. This is not a bad thing because it at least gets the patient talking about something, and communicating with another person. What you can do as a caregiver is show the patient photographs of the events they are talking about that happened to them in the past. These photographs can easily be a trigger to get them to start talking any time you want them to. So if you think they have been too quiet lately,

34

then pull out some photographs and show them to the patient. This should get them to open up again. The more they communicate, the more they will be exercising their brain function and will practice their socializing skills. In some cases, it may even get patients to talk more than they usually do and trust their caregiver. This is your main goal here.

If you come across a patient that doesn't want to talk about anything, then you as the caregiver must start the conversation. Just make the topic about the past, especially the patient's childhood. Ask the patient about where they went to school or what kind of job they used to have. Then to engage the discussion you can tell them about your parents and what jobs they used to have back in the day. As long as you are talking about past experiences of the patient or someone else, it will take their minds off their condition. But if for some reason the patient starts talking about their condition, be prepared for an emotional outburst. Some patients have trouble being distracted from the pain while others have an easier time. The ones who get distracted are going to be the hardest to talk to. In such cases, the best thing you can do is show empathy towards their situation. Never talk down upon them or make them feel like they are a burden on you or their families. That kind of talk will definitely send them over the edge. Instead, remind them of the good things they still have in their lives and the loving family they have who comes to see them often.

The severe cases of dementia can be real trouble in the communication department. Those deeply affected by dementia won't say a word or won't even respond to a visual form of communication, like photos and art. You could even try playing music, but they'll act like they don't even hear it because their mind is so far gone in their imaginations. In these extreme cases, touch communication is all that is left. Touch creates more of a feeling in the person than anything else. You should only lightly touch your patients on the hands or shoulders to create this feeling. Do not push or shake the patients because that would almost be considered as abuse. Instead, light touches on the hand or shoulders are a way of showing compassion and empathy towards their condition. Those who have enough brain function to appreciate that will likely give you a smile or some other kind of facial expression as a response. However, there are some dementia patients that don't like to be touched, but these are usually the ones that can speak and are quick to complain about it. With those patients, just use the other forms of communication you have learned to get them to open up.

Independence

One of the most important things you can do for a dementia patient is to make them feel like they are independent. The dementia condition has already taken away the patient's freedom to care for themselves the way they used to, which causes depression on top of all the other psychological symptoms that go along with it. This means they need to have opportunities to care for themselves without a caregiver doing everything for them. The activities you coordinate will help them feel independent as long as you let them do as much of the work as possible. Caregivers are only the moderators and guides of their patients.

Dementia patients need to get into an active routine of performing activities that benefit themselves. These can be everyday activities like getting dressed, bathing, folding clothes and brushing their teeth. As a caregiver, you just need to make sure they do them. But whatever you do, don't do those chores for them unless they are physically unable to. For example, a dementia patient that has short term memory loss will still have the capacity to cook their foods and do their laundry. They just have to be reminded to do them because they will forget. Your job as a caregiver is to simply remind them and to possibly leave the materials out that will help them do this. With everything laid out in front of them, they can do the work without forgetting anything. Of course, make sure you are nearby in case they run into trouble and need assistance. But as long as they feel like they are doing it, their sense of independence will be there.

Patients should not be left alone if they suffer from moderate to severe dementia. If they have mild dementia, they should still be monitored everyday to see how worse their condition has gotten because dementia only gets worse as time goes on. Nobody gets stuck in mild or moderate stages of dementia forever. In the end, they all end up suffering from severe dementia. At the same time, you have to give them all as much independence as possible. The mild cases of dementia will get the most freedom because they won't have caregivers living with them and coordinating their activities every day.

But the more serious cases will require either a professional caregiver or a family member to watch over the patient carefully and even live with them. They won't necessarily sleep in the same room, but they will sleep in the same house and have a monitoring device to hear the noises in the patient's room. It is hard to give independence to a patient with severe dementia, but try to do the best you can with it.

Conclusion

Dementia is a condition that makes life more challenging than it already is. You could try taking all the medications and prescription drugs that you want, but nothing is going to replace the feeling of losing your independence and ability to perform physical activity. These are things that all people value in their lives, whether they have dementia or not. But for dementia patients, it is even more important they feel active and self dependent because it keeps their confidence levels high and they don't lose hope. In so many cases of dementia, people often refrain from performing activities because they feel too depressed about their situation. That is why it is important that their family and friends get involved in their treatment by encouraging them to do more activities.

There are so many books on dementia out on the market, but very few of them emphasize the importance of activities. Instead, they focus on prescription medications because they know the quick and easy solution always sells on the market. This creates a false mindset in people by making them think something as serious as dementia can be treated by just popping a pill in your mouth once a day. The truth is that no problem in life can be cured by popping pills. It takes action and motivation to really make a change in your life for the better. For a dementia patient, it takes action towards activities that take their mind off their problems and get them interested in something again. Other books on the market may casually touch upon this subject and say activities help, but you have to understand that activities do more than just help. They are, in fact, the only treatment that effectively helps dementia patients lead happier lives.

I hope you have found this book helpful. If you have read the entire book then chances are you or a loved one is suffering from dementia and you were seeking guidance on how to deal with it. After you have experimented with the advice given to you in this book, I would love it if you left me a review on Amazon to show your appreciation. Dementia is a never ending battle that needs to be constantly fought. Together, we can all fight the battle and help our loved ones who are caught in the middle.

Good luck to you all!
THANK YOU!

Made in the USA
Middletown, DE
21 January 2018